CASTLEBERRY HEALTH SOLUTIONS PRESENTS

LIVING LIKE WATER

MY ESCAPE FROM THE ACID PIT

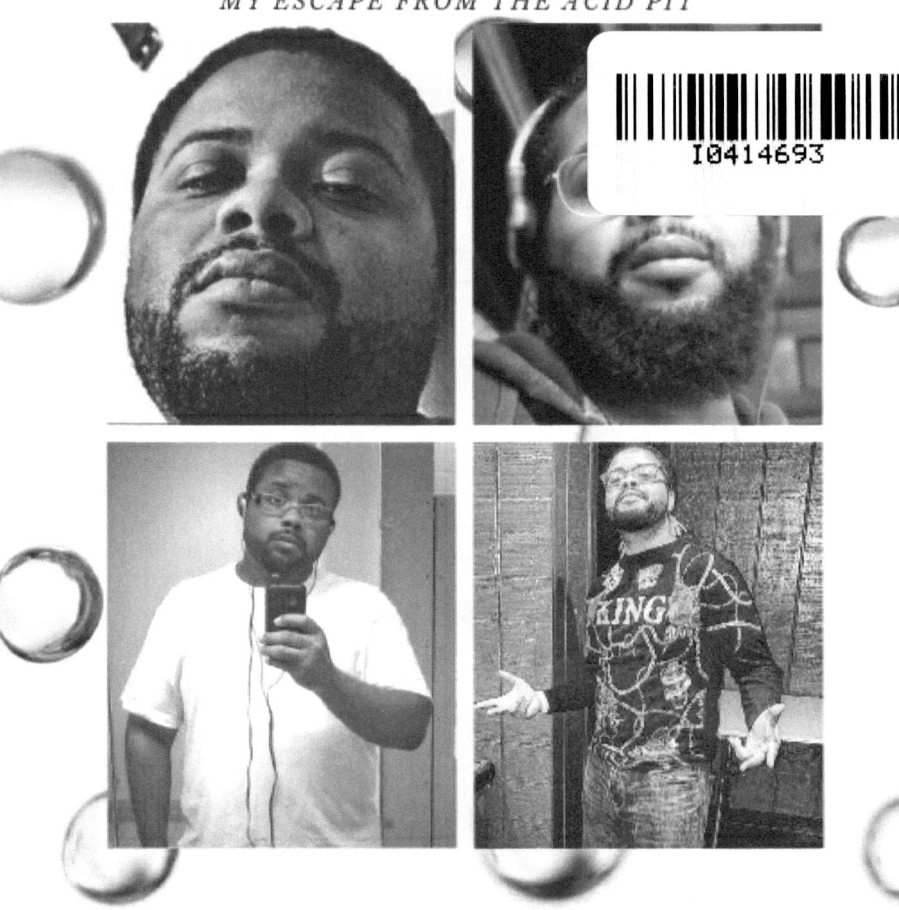

I0414693

D.M. CASTLEBERRY

LIVING LIKE WATER:

My Escape From The Acid Pit

D. M. Castleberry

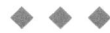

Castleberry Health Solutions 2019

I wrote this in honor of my mother Sheryl Lynn Upton. She taught me that I could be whatever I wanted to be. I hope I can always honor my family and lead them to any treasure that I find. A journey is less fun without people to celebrate it with...

- Dwayne M. Castleberry

Mucus is the cause of every disease. Eliminate the mucus and you eliminate the disease

- DR. SEBI

People don't want to change their diets, I get that. But if you don't want to change your diet, enjoy your suffering. Man just hasn't come to understand, how vital his diet is.

- DR. ROBERT MORSE

I'M JUST A REGULAR GUY

Hey, I'm Dwayne, a Libra that likes to travel. I also like long walks on the beach. Sorry, I couldn't help it. All joking aside, my name is Dwayne Castleberry. I'm a graphic designer, performance artist, activist, public speaker, and owner of Castleberry Health Solutions. Yeah, thats alot, but hold on folks, that's not all. I am a studio engineer and mentor many artists. I have a bit of an obsession with learning. It became a habit of mine to disappeared from public life just to study. I've never been a stranger to a library and have read through hundreds of books. If they weren't comic books, they were books that taught you something. That was a trait given to me from my mother who had self-help and how-to books all throughout the house that we grew up in. I was always top percentile of my classes, along with the top percentile of knuckleheads. You will rarely hear me tooting my own whistle, but I want you to get closer to knowing the author so that you can understand my approach more clearly.

I was always ahead of my class in academics. Surprisingly, that made me a horrible student. My arrogance about my knowledge made me miss the point of school. It was to learn a system and I didn't want to learn it. It was boring and couldn't keep my attention which led me to dropping out. I eventually went back for a degree a couple years later, but I could have received it much earlier. That was just one of my life lessons that taught me that sometimes you have to do things that you don't want to do to get where you want to get. Changing how we eat is the same way. In my personal experience, people usually don't want to adjust their diet unless for religious/spiritual rites, poverty or to improve an health issue. I believe many of us are suffering from an widespread health issue. I've found a cure.

I am not a millionaire nutritionist with infomercials and some wacky pill that will make you a superman or wonder woman. I'm just a guy that had an obsession with knowledge that led me to losing half my body weight. I tried all of the popular diets and none of them worked. I tried starving myself, but that just made me a ravenous beast. I tried to just not care and 2 months later I was 50 lbs heavier. I just couldn't figure it out. Maybe its just in my genes. Hold on...I wouldn't be writing this book if I didn't figure it out.

In the following chapters I will go over my journey from a 285 lb dead man walking to an mix between a chiseled god and a 160 lb average Joe. I will start off with why I started this journey and why it means so much to me. I will go over some of my ups and downs in hopes that it will save you from repeating them again. P.S. you will. I will also talk about the treasure...my precious. I won't do you like the golem. I'm not a troll either. In fact, I want to lead you to the fountain of life. Most people fear the fountain of life because it requires sacrifice. Put the goat back...not that type of sacrifice. Let's talk about it more. Take my hand...you don't have to be weird about it.

I DIDN'T KNOW I WAS A FAT KID

I have broken the secret code to the human body and I'm selling it for a billion dollars. Is that too much for you...okay, you can just pay the Amazon price and owe me. My health and well-being has always been on my mind, but I found out the hard way, that it didn't equal being healthy. As a kid, my brothers would pick on me because of my picky eating habits. I would just eat the less fatty parts of the meat, leaving half of it on the plate. My parents would tell me to finish my plate, but my body would not let me do it. I took a couple ol'skool L's for it(I got my behind whooped). I didn't like vegetables either, unless they were french fried or covered in glorious sacred cheese. The end result was a very unbalanced diet that consisted mostly of lunch meat, fried chicken, pork chops, and whatever processed goodies I could get my hands on. I could take out a family bag of skittles in one sitting and it showed on me.

I didn't know I was a fat kid until my school days. I was a little guy and most of my family is "big boned" so there was no issue with extra pounds. I actually believed it was just a phase of life. In my world, once you were old enough, the magical cellulite fairies would come and bless you with the sacred pounds. Just like clockwork, the pounds started to pack on around 3rd grade. My youthful metabolism would have me changing weight often but most of the time, I was a hefty kid. The jokes came often and I was known as the fat kid or the big butt kid.

All the jokes were pretty harsh and led me to become a very defensive person. I had no problem sending jokes back because of my sense of humor, but if I got mad enough, then we had to fight. Most of my childhood fights were from jokers trying to make me the highlight of their impromptu stand-up routine. I was notching off a few victories but it was not a healthy way to deal with things. After awhile I started to internalize many of the comments and started to doubt my appearance. Hormones kicked in and I started to notice the love handles and man-boobs a little bit more. The extra weight was already there and a natural part of me, but the jokes just really got to me. The media's hate for fat, didn't help. It felt like all I had to rely on was my personality, so I took it to the extreme.

KEEPING UP WITH THE (6) PACK

The world didn't take long to let me know that I was a fat kid and it hurt. According to TV, the fat kid sucked and was only good for comic relief. My fears were verified by me google searching "the fat kid from…". All the famous fat kid characters popped up. The one that stuck out was one from one of my favorite movies, Goonies. The fat kid, who was literally named "Chunk", played by actor Jeff Cohen, was just constantly made fun of in the movie. He even did a fat dance that became popular called the "truffle shuffle". The dance consisted of him lifting his shirt and shaking his belly. This is what I had to look forward too. I should not have been trying to model myself from a movie character anyway, but I was a kid.

The character Chunk, was made fun of by others, but what was his approach? For the most it seemed like he would just roll with the jokes, but as mentioned in the prior section, I was too much of a fighter to just be somebody's punchline. I had a few jokes, but wasn't funny enough to be the funny big guy. The younger me was caught between judging the heavier people around me, and following Hollywood stereotypes. I was a kid trying to find where to fit in and I had to learn. Chunk would also make up stories to fit in. He would use his communication and manipulation to maintain some form of status within the group. I wasn't much of a liar so the answer for me was to use my communication skills to become extra charming. I needed something to keep up with the six-pack guys so my journey to build myself began.

My first stop was the library. I read daily about psychology, public speaking, relationships, and history. I learned about etiquette and other things that I felt would bring me closer to becoming the perfect person. The journey was so amazing. Reading and writing became a daily routine. Sharing poetry and music became a passion. By the time high-school came around, I was a renaissance man, The problem was I was still dealing with some old demons.

In my pursuit for perfection, I learned many things, including the fact that I wasn't happy. I was considered a weird kid compared to other kids my age. They were playing tag, while little Dwayne was reading about the theory of relativity. They were playing with water guns, I was laying in a pile of encyclopedias learning about the life around me. They were playing and having fun, my mind was worried about the economy and the threat of nuclear war(I hadn't even hit puberty yet). To make a long story short, I was so focused on becoming perfect, that I was missing many little things, mainly how to be a kid(very important). All my knowledge did not hide the fat feeling. It didn't stop the man boob jokes.

It's pretty sad, but don't worry there is a happy ending. I had to hit rock bottom. You may have to hit rock bottom also but hopefully my struggles can help you avoid some of the same pain. I remember sitting in my bedroom with a shotgun(whole other story) thinking about how bad my life was. The negative things in my life had finally overwhelmed my mind. I stuck the barrel under my chin and closed my eyes. In that moment nothing else mattered but the pain in currently my life. In that moment Dwayne was the fat loser. Luckily a moment of clarity hit me as I began to see the faces of my family and friends. I felt like a fool. There were so many great things going on in my life, but I chose to make the bad things prominent. Some things weren't bad, my vision was just clouded. The shotgun dropped to the floor and started my life over with a new focus. My focus became to be the best me.

Let's not forget Jeff Cohen. After he hit puberty and lost

the extra weight, he actually struggled because of his new body. Hollywood didn't hire him anymore, because he no longer had the weight to be the fat comedic relief. The public's desire to laugh at fat folks left no place for Jeff Cohen's dream of being an actor. He didn't let the rejection destroy him though. Instead he studied at UCLA and became an entertainment lawyer for Universal Studios Television. So be encouraged my chunky angels, you are more than your body type.

At any time things can get overwhelming. Tomorrow can seem like too much, but we don't know. We just don't know. When you don't know something, all you can do is learn or prepare to your best ability. Any preconceived notion about an unknown thing isn't real. It's literally just your imagination. Your imagination can be used to hype you up for a situation or it can scare you right out of one. Okay, I know this is a health book, and we might be digging into philosophy, but I want you to understand that it's going to take a change in your mindset to form a habit. We want your habit to be a healthy lifestyle.

FAILED DIETS

The main thing you need to learn to do is lose. Of course you want to lose weight, but you will also have to lose the parts of your mindset that led you into an unhealthy lifestyle. Lose the expectations of the television diets. Many are fad based and over-hype one segment of a system, such as carbs or calories. I have tried many, and failed at many.

My first method was to starve myself. That didn't last long. My portions were so small I'm surprised that my plates weren't flying away. The weight just wouldn't leave. It might have had something to do with the late night creeps. You know the late night creeps. The lack of food and nutrition would turn me into a zombie looking for junk food. It would usually be something like fried lunch meat drizzled in cheese, fried again in bread and butter, with a side of ice cream, potato chips, skittles, Reese's cups, some super sweet Kool-aid and whatever else my hands could find. I actually thought my diet was healthy. Heck, I would just starve it off the next day which turned me into the walking fed- (get it… whatever, that was funny).

My food zombie days were long and still affect me till this day. I have to actively tell myself to eat sometimes. The body craves what it wants but it lives off what it needs. During those days, I was sick often, mostly colds and the flu. Allergies would take over the rest of the time. My weight was up and my energy was low. Things had to change.

My next major diet change was protein based. Even though I wasn't the healthiest, I grew up around many athletes. Some who made it to play sports professionally. So I would go on work out binges. Everybody would tell me, eat alot of protein to lose weight. Eat so much protein that you sweat it. A steak a day keeps the doctor away (away from other patients so that they can tend to you).

My diet consisted of a big meaty breakfast with many sides. Lunch was usually a multi-meat monster sandwich with chips/dip and a little Debbie cake or 2 or maybe 3. My mother was known for making big dinners. She had 3 big boys and a small one who could eat just like them.

My muscles started to grow with my new diet and work-out plan. I actually got a little bulky under my fat. My fat was getting bulky over my muscle also. My body had spurts of energy but would go through dead battery moments. Dead battery moments were those times when my body would just shut down rather I did something physical or not. My system needed sleep instantly in the middle of the day. I wasn't only physically tired, but I was so exhausted that my thinking process was cloudy.

My energy levels were a mess and I noticed that it was lowest mostly after eating. This was crazy because I was taught that food was fuel for the body. So why was I losing energy from food? Folks were telling me that's it normal, it's just the itis. The itis is not normal, turns out it takes alot of energy to break down the excessive protein. At the time I attributed the bad protein to red meat, so I just gave it up and stuck with poultry and seafood.

After giving up red meat my energy went up and my weight went down. Giving up soda and other soft drinks in exchange for more water helped also. The very physical factory job I had helped as part of my workout. Combined with jogging every other day, my routine was pretty solid. I was running circles around my coworkers because I had a physical goal to achieve. I began to lose 1-2lbs on average a week until I got down to 180 lbs. Yep, 100lbs gone.

People were amazed at the dramatic change in my appearance. In a few months I had lost about a third of my body weight and had to buy a completely new wardrobe. Many people didn't even recognize me anymore. That caused many awkward moments.

Everything was good until an unexpected change of jobs.

I went from lifting and dumping 60 lbs bags 12 hours a day to a desk job. My weight came back as fast as it left. I joined a few workout classes to stop the weight gain but nothing could stop the return of my big belly and boobies. Before I knew it, my weight was back up to 230lbs. I couldn't believe it and it made me give up. I completely gave up.

TIME TO FIND THE REAL ISSUE?

I started attending Cleveland State University and it changed my life. A healthy diet wasn't on my mind anymore so it was time to indulge in every restaurant possible in downtown Cleveland. I was living the college life. Pizza, chicken wings, and subs became the main foods in my diet. On top of that, my relationship with the folks running the school buffet meant free food. I was also a member of many campus organizations which meant more free food.

The free food helped me through many hard times but it did nothing good for my health. There was one voice of reason, Jake Streeter, who was the only vegetarian in our circle, who would speak many dietary warnings that we all ignored mostly. We will get back to that. My health declined badly and I definitely noticed it. Something had to be done. I was in college so I did what we were taught to do...study.

I was always told that being big was a family trait. It was believable. I could physically see that there were many heavy set family members. But what about the skinny family members? Did they sneak a skinny gene in from extended bloodlines? Did their parents marry into skinny? What about my little brother?

While me and my two older brothers were chubby kids my little brother was a skinny kid. I also have cousins that have like 0 percent body fat, which meant that genes couldn't be blamed for the size of my jeans. Instead what I observed was that we were a group of people who basically have the same eating habits. It affected most of us the same with a few exceptions. After eliminating genes as a cause, human anatomy was the next step. Time to see what humans are built to eat.

Patterns can be seen throughout nature. We study those patterns and make classifications such as carnivores and herbivores. From observing many carnivores or meat eating animals, a person can observe similarities such as big, sharp canine teeth. These animals usually have a natural weapon on them such as sharp claws or venom. People have none of these characteristics. We don't have the agility of a chimp, we don't have the speed of a cheetah, We don't have the strength of a lion. A snail has more defenses than we do. We don't have camouflage like the predators of the sea or wings and talons of sky hunters. We are actually like the least physically impressive beings on the planet.

One of the first things observable from most animals is their teeth. I looked at carnivores and no teeth were similar to humans. The biggest difference being large sharp canines that they need to tear at flesh and shells. Other animals have completely alien mouths like sharks who can have rows of sharp teeth. Omnivores were a little closer to humans because they have molars for eating plants but they still had carnivore type canines that we don't have. I look at herbivores and they have flat molars for chewing plants. Most had small canines or none at all. Sound familiar? This perfectly describes the mouth of a human.

It was shocking what I learned about teeth but It didn't make me give up meat right away. I did immediately start eating more veggies with my meals. My studies weren't over either. The next study was the digestive system. I mean it is where food goes after the teeth rip it apart.

The study of the digestive system was short but complicated because within mammals exist many adaptations, but still certain digestive organs in these animals stuck very closely to the teeth type. The carnivores with the big canines had very short intestines and their big stomachs makes up most of their highly acidic digestive system. Their stomach acid is 10 times the acidity of a human. They need this acid to break down and extract the nutrients from the dense meat.

The herbivores and many omnivores had smaller stomachs and longer intestines with the exception of the weird stomachs of grazing animals such as cows and deer. Humans definitely have smaller stomachs in comparison to our intestines which can stretch around the world. Ha! I'm joking. I know we all heard that as a kid. In all honestly the human intestines stretch to around 25 feet. Our stomachs average about a foot long and 6 inches wide. That fits the small stomach, long intestines requirement of herbivores and some omnivores. Even though I grew up as meat being the main course, I couldn't see any evidence that it was part of our natural diet. I added more veggies and fruits to my diet and cut down more on the meat. My studies continued.

LEARNING TO LIVE LIKE WATER

One particular semester at Cleveland State University a classmate suggested that I sign up for a class called Cleveland Natural History. The class was amazing for a nature guy like me. It taught me so much about the things around me everyday. I didn't know I walked past witch hazel trees all the time in gritty ol' Cleveland Ohio. My final was a presentation about dead lakes. I studied hard and what I found was amazing.

First off, a dead lake or pond is a body of water that has accumulated so much acidic waste that it can't support life anymore. The pH level of the water becomes so low that it will literally cook any fish in it. If you didn't know, pH levels measure the level of acidity and alkalinity. The lower the pH the more acidic. The water in the pond becomes undrinkable and dangerous for most life on earth. The cause is dead plants and animals that have decomposed at a high level for an extended amount of time. The lightbulb became so bright in my head when I learned this.

Let me break it down. The human body is about 45 to 65 percent water depending on weight and height. It only made sense that anything that changes the life giving qualities of water should directly affect at least 45 to 65 percent of a person's health. So if dead matter kills the life giving qualities of water then it has to take life from us also. Our systems aren't made like the lions'. Meat stays in our stomach. As meat lingers in our system it decomposes just like the roadkill on the side of the road. Ugh. The stinky smells and putridness of a rotting animal is all there sitting in your stomach along with whatever parasite or worm that comes with it. The human body amps up its acidity but it's not enough. The water that flows through our blood becomes like the water in the dead pond. Our bodies become so acidic that it literally begins to digest itself.

With a system full of acid, the body begins to inflame and produce excessive mucus to protect itself. The part of the body that inflames determines what illnesses we encounter. In its most basic form, colds and influenza are swelling of the respiratory system and excess mucus. The body does this to fight whatever issue it has encountered. Many other illnesses such as bronchitis have the same symptoms. In fact it wouldn't be hard to show that almost every non-bacterial illness is tracked to the inflammation of either the respiratory, digestive, or circulatory system. This process is normal and would work to keep us healthy, but many don't allow their bodies to recover. Meat leaves our bodies in a constant state of detoxification which doesn't allow meat eaters to ever be in a state of stable health. The body treats the meat stuck in our intestines similar to a virus. If meat is part of your main diet, your body is in overdrive right now trying to normalize your system.

On the other hand, when we eat plants, our digestive system is allowed to do its work. First our molars grind the plants and our saliva breaks it down more to extract the first round of nutrients. This is our natural juicing system. Many nutrients are absorbed before they ever reach the stomach. The next stage is the stomach where the plants enter into a pool of acid. This acid extracts most of the remaining nutrients and dispels the remaining fiber. This fiber makes its way through the intestines where even more nutrients are collected. The fiber also does double duty to clean any food waste left behind from the last meal. Anything that wasn't used by the body is then released by sweat, acne, and when we use the restroom. This is why a meat eating person may experience stomach discomfort when they eat more plants.

Since meat can't be digested properly, it is caking up inside the intestines. The fiber from the plants begins to clear it out. This causes discolored and smelly boo boo. I definitely experienced it personally. The first thing I experienced was some wicked gas that could clear a room. I would try to duck off and escape when I felt one bubbling up, but some folks just had to take the funk. Okay back to the adult stuff. Make sure you drink water. I should have said that in the beginning. Drink water. Again, I personally experienced this. If you don't drink water during your transformation into a plant-based diet, you will most likely get constipation. You should see the difference inside the toilet. In the beginning your bowel movements may be a dance between discolored loose stool to longer solid stool. This is normal because your body is detoxing. Over time your bowel movements will become smaller and more consistent as the fiber and plant minerals clean the waste out of your digestive system. Sorry, I know that was graphic but the digestive system is the main part of the journey to optimal health.

DEAR MEAT, I LOVE YOU BUT I GOTTA GO

I did some deep soul searching and made the decision to give up meat all together. It started to become easier because of Jake Streeter, whom I mentioned earlier. I was president of the Speak Up Poetry Slam Organization at the time. Jake is an amazing poet, who won our poetry slams often. His vegetarian ways forced us to change our menu, so I just followed his lead. By the way, Jake is also a public speaker and founder of MIE Life Now a youth mentoring program in Cleveland, Ohio. Check him out.

I figured my last stand against meat should be a buffet. I tried a little of everything as my goodbye to meat. A lil steak here, a lil shrimp and chicken there. The main course was a big ol' mountain of bacon. Nothing else, just bacon. After a couple bites I just thought in my head that this crap is disgusting. I threw the Mt. Everest of bacon right in the garbage and left.

With the meat gone, I just began to feel so much better. I had so much more energy. The fat on my body just began to melt away. I wasn't even working out. My job and my business both required me to sit in front of computers for long periods of time so I wasn't very active. It didn't matter, the weight just flew away. I would hit the gym maybe once or twice a month. The excessive calories and fat just wasn't in my diet anymore so my body slimmed down. Now remember I was around 230 beforehand, but I was now down to 180 lbs. At this point, anybody who knew me was amazed at my transformation. Some wouldn't even recognize me unless we talked. I was happy. I set a goal and my efforts were being shown to the world. I had an old buddy try to come and wreck my party though.

I had full confidence in my studies and I could visually see it everyday. It wasn't like the other diets. I felt the best that I could remember feeling but I was still addicted to chicken. The smell of it would bring back childhood memories of my mother cooking dinner. Y'all know that smell that fried chicken lets off. That smell throws hunger into overdrive. Some restaurants even fan the smell out to attract customers and trust me, it works. I was addicted, I probably still am. The smell still stimulates my hunger. I started back eating chicken maybe once every couple weeks. Then I started working banquet events.

Chicken and pork were definitely the most served foods at the banquet events I worked. The chicken was cooked in so many fancy ways, but the only vegan option was iceberg salad. I hate iceberg lettuce. Most veggies were just garnish or cooked with the meat. There was fruit salad sometimes, but at that time I was still afraid of the sugar in fruit. I chose to indulge in the chicken. It was like my survival instincts overpowered my knowledge. Well, not really, it was more like my bank account said eat what you can or starve. The food at the job was catered and free of charge. The choice was hard for my new life journey, but very easy for my pockets. The problem was that it seemed like many times my choices would be between just some garnish or some chef-prepared Chicken with some rosemary wine sauce or something. I chose the fancy option.

My step back into the carnivorous world had its consequences. I started to have stomach problems instantly and often. My weight tried to creep its way back up also. I was down to 170 lbs but went right back up to 180 lbs. I felt the effects physically and mentally. The clarity that I had gained was leaving me.

LIVING LIKE WATER

While I was battling with my chicken addiction, I was also expanding my knowledge of the human diet. The study of pH levels in the dead ponds stuck with me. High acidity kills the functionality of water. We are water-based beings therefore high acidity kills the functionality of humans. The natural cycle of the water get disturbed by excess animal/plant waste which ferments or decomposes which raises the level of acidity. This kills the filtering process. This makes the lake/pond toxic to most forms of life. The human equivalent would be the digestive system. We feed the digestive system and the digestive system feeds the rest of the body. That is key to understanding this philosophy young grasshopper.

Everything we eat is filtered so our bodies can process it. Just like the lake, if our filters aren't working right, the waste will accumulate. Waste accumulation equals acid. Acid burns us and our body reacts to survive. Our body has three major reactions to injury or intoxication, swelling(inflammation), snot(mucus), and pus(pimples,boils). All of these are methods of healing, but imagine having a ongoing body cold/flu that won't go away. If you eat meat that's basically what's happening to your body. Its nature.

Man, I had trouble spreading my message. I didn't know of any scholars that would back my theory and personal findings. I started to research but couldn't find much. The closest thing I found was a video of an amazing guy named Dr. Sebi. I can't remember the exact video because I've watched a few at this point, but I do remember he was talking about the body being electric. He had a similar but more seasoned view on eating meat and pH levels than me. I felt like I had a kindred spirit that I would never meet. I learned how important herbs are for healing the body from his lectures. Dr. Sebi's video lectures, along with a few others like Aqiyl Aniys, and Robert Morse help helped fill in so much details of my current knowledge on the human body. Make sure you check out their stuff.

The healing nature of fruits and herbs is amazing. They are literally the cure to most illness. There are documented cases of HIV and and cancer being cured through an alkaline diet. Dr. Sebi even successfully defended his claims of curing multiple diseases in court. The judge asked that he provide a witness for every disease that he had cured. The judge dismissed the case when 77 people showed up.

I was so happy about putting this knowledge together that I tried to tell everyone I knew. I had a few different reactions from people including some that blew my mind. Some would congratulate me and conclude that it was just my thing. In my mind I thought that this was a human thing. Chicken was my thing, but I couldn't ignore what nature was showing me.

Many people had concerns about the sugar in fruits. Fruit sugar was meant to be the main source of energy for humans. Most processed sugars are bad and lead to many ailments. If nature didn't grow it, then chances are that your body can't naturally digest it. Most fruit sugars won't raise insulin levels like the processed counterparts. Although it doesn't affect you the same, you should still try to have a good balance of low-fructose and high-fructose fruits. Just look at it like this, high-fructose means high energy which is good for the morning. In contrast low-fructose is better for mid-day.

Others would spark up a debate/argument. I mean some folks would get so mad that I gave up meat. I just didn't understand it. It's not like I was going door to door spreading my message of veggie salvation. Most of these confrontations came from either someone seeing me eat or someone asking me about food. It became so repetitive that I would try to avoid the conversations. I've been yelled at and called out my name. I wish my testimonial was that I handled all those situations perfectly, but I didn't. It was frustrating at first but I was down to 160 lbs and feeling better than I could remember so nothing was going to stop me...

This is the end of the book but it is just the beginning of this amazing series. This introduction was meant to build a foundation. The next books in this series will include detailed fruit and herbs list, recipes, and motivation tips.

Follow us on Instagram @CastleberryHealth to stay updated. Like us on Facebook also. Email us   CastleberryHealth@gmail.com

Castleberry Health Solutions 2019

www.ingramcontent.com/pod-product-compliance
Lightning Source LLC
Chambersburg PA
CBHW020333290526
45785CB00007B/3045